God Speaks to Us Through Dreams and Visions

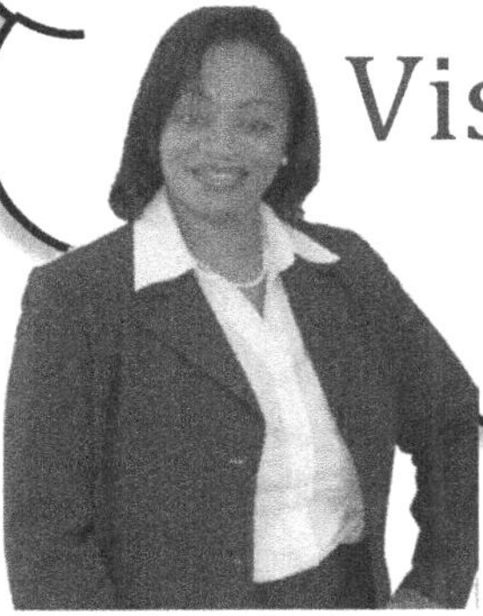

GOD Did It!

By

Janet Green

"[14]For God speaketh once,
yea twice, yet man perceiveth it not.
[15]In a dream, in a vision of the night, when deep
sleep falleth upon men, in slumberings upon the bed;"

Job 33: 14-15 KJV

Olmstead Publishing LLC

GOD Did It!

God Speaks to Us Through Dreams and Visions

By Janet Green
Janet@GodWills.com
www.facebook.com/Talent2business
www.facebook.com/GodSpeaksToUsThroughDreamsAndVisions

Cover and Formatting by Dr Phyllis M Olmstead

Olmstead Publishing LLC
www.olmsteadpublishing.com
OlmsteadPublishing@usa.com
www.facebook.com/OlmsteadPublishing

All biblical quotations are from the King James Version (KJV).

Thoughts

Thought clouds are provided throughout this book so that you may jot down or drawn ideas and questions as you read and implement the material presented.

Table of Contents

Introduction to Dreams and Visions

Does God speak to us through dreams and visions?

As far as back I can remember, I have always had dreams. I thought it was a special gift, not knowing that God speaks to everyone through dreams. In this chapter, I will help you understand the importance of paying attention to your dreams, and realizing that, in most cases, it is God who is communicating to us through dreams and visions.

It is exciting to know that God is our personal coach and He is giving direction, guidance, and gifts to us in our dreams. It is up to us to pay attention, and respond according to what God is instructing us to do. Remember it is God's will for us to be prosperous in all areas of our lives. As simple as it may sound, the most difficult part of this process is to act upon what God instructs us to do.

For those of you who do not believe that you are dreaming at night, I will give you some basic principles on how to activate your dream relationship with God. Once you believe that God speaks to you through dreams and visions you will start to have more dreams. I also will teach you how to journal your dreams. What is so significant about our dreams is that they usually speak to us in regards to current and future situations. How awesome it is to get a peak of what God has in store for us.

Yes, Satan can also give you dreams. We will discuss how to recognize when a dream is from God or from Satan.

Once you begin to have dreams more frequently, you will develop a hunger to have them interpreted. ALWAYS remember dream interpretation belongs to God. **Genesis 40:8 King James Version (KJV)** [8]*And they said unto him, We have dreamed a dream, and there is no interpreter of it. And, Joseph said unto them, Do not interpretations belong to God? Tell me them, I pray you.*

Therefore, you should apply biblical principles when interpreting your dreams. Pray before you attempt to interpret your dreams. Let the Holy Spirit take control and let God work through you to give you an accurate interpretation of your dream.

We will discuss later the different ways that God gives us interpretations of our dreams. In addition, knowing the different types of dreams you will receive from God will help during the interpretation process.

You do not want to miss the opportunity of having dream and vision encounters with God. They will change your life forever. Do you know that it is God's desire to speak to us through dreams and visions? I will teach you in this chapter how to activate a relationship with God so that you begin to hear Him through your dreams.

An aside for those readers who are implementing my program, ***How to Turn Your Talent into a Business***:

What do dreams and visions have to do with building a business?

I am glad you asked. Since the business you plan to start came from God as a part of His will for your life, don't you want His guidance through the entire process?

Okay, let us explore this chapter together.

What are Dreams and Visions?

Numbers 12:6 KJV [6]And he said, Hear now my words: If there be a prophet among you, I the LORD will make myself known unto him in a vision, and will speak unto him in a dream.

Therefore, we can say that God will make himself known to us in a vision. He will talk to us. His instruction will be much clearer and easier to understand than a dream.

God promised to speak to us in dreams. We see throughout the *Bible* that God speaks in parables. Therefore, we know dreams will be a little more difficult to understand. However, because dream interpretation belongs to God and its God's desire for us to understand Him when he speaks to us, then all we have to do is pray and ask Him to help us interpret our dreams.

Thoughts

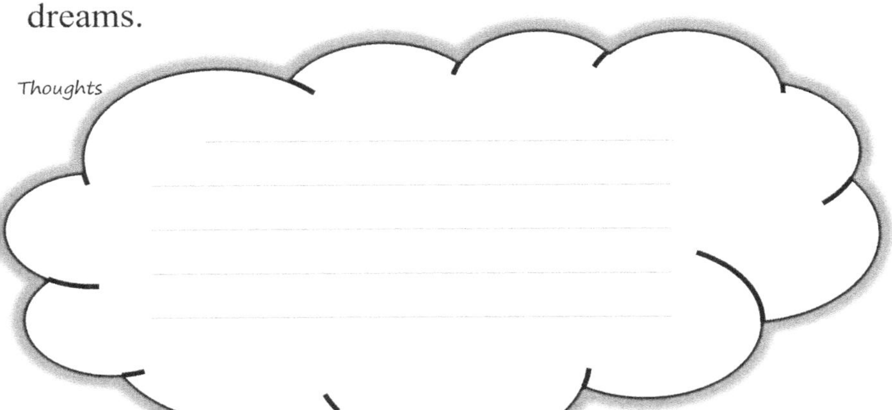

How to Strengthen Your Communication with God through Dreams and Visions

Every one of us dreams at night. Some of us remember our dreams and others do not. We often disregard dreams because we think they are insignificant. Appling the following principles will help you recall your dreams and discover how important they are.

A. Pray and ask God to speak to you through dreams and visions. Ask God's forgiveness because you ignored Him all the years He has been speaking to you.

Remember the saying "So a man thinketh so is he" also, Job 22:28 28*Thou shalt also decree a thing, and it shall be established unto thee.* We have the power to speak things into existence. We have to renew the way we thing about dreams, therefore speaking aloud with sincerity saying, "I believe in dreams and visions because it's a mean of communication from God. Dreams and visions have vital messages from God to me and I will pay attention to them."

B. Put a notepad (i.e., journal, diary) and a pen on your nightstand beside your bed so that you can record your dreams upon awakening. Do not procrastinate recording your dreams, as you will forget them. Write them down immediately upon awakening.

C. Title and date your dreams. See the sample in the back of this book.

D. Record the time you woke up from your dream as biblical scriptures may support the meaning of your dream based upon the time.

E. Avoid using an alarm clock to wake up, as this will often frighten you from your sleep and will often cause you to forget your dream.

F. Try not to fall asleep while watching television as this could contribute to your dreams.

G. Try to fall asleep naturally; do not take sleeping pills or alcohol to fall asleep.

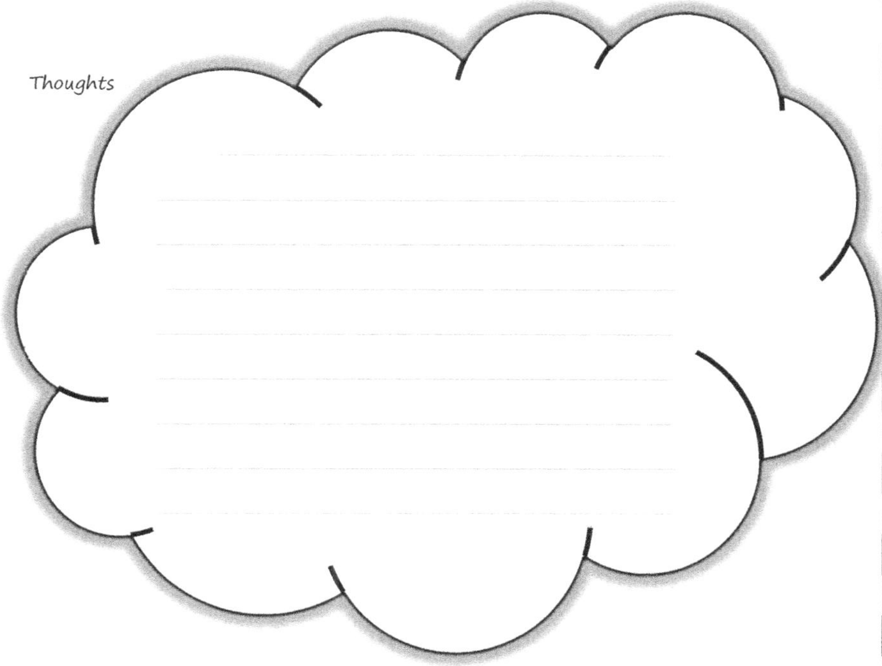

Paying Attention to Your Dreams and Visions Can Help You Live a Fulfilling Life

In 2009, I prayed and asked God to close all doors that should be closed and open all doors that needed to be open in my life. Little did I know how powerfully that prayer would affect my life and that it would transition me from a 20-year career to volunteering as a director of the Entrepreneur Ministry at my home church.

It did not make sense to me to make such a transition until I had a vision from God. That vision gave me peace of mind as I moved into the ministry leadership role. Even though this was on a voluntarily basis, I was much happier than working as an executive with a six-figure income. God knows what He created us to do, therefore if we seek His guidance when we make decisions in life we will live a more fulfilling life.

It is very important that we set the foundation by inviting God into our lives. Staying in constant communication (praying, fasting, reading His words and meditating on his words) with God. God wants to be a part of our lives. God will not force Himself on us. We have free will but once we invite Him in you will be amaze how often he will communicate to us through dreams, visions, and others. You have to do your part by make sure that your communication line with Him is open. He is our creator, He knows us better than we know our selves.

Reasons why we should pay attention to our Dreams and Visions

God is our creator therefore, He knows us more than we know ourselves. If you have a mechanical problem with a new car, you take it to the manufacture for a diagnostic test and you follow their instructions on what to do to resolve the issue.

A. Is God giving us directions for our businesses, where to go to start our business? God gives directions in dream; Matthew 2:12-13 King James Version (KJV) [12]*And being warned of God in a dream that they should not return to Herod, they departed into their own country another way.* [13]*And when they were departed, behold, the angel of the Lord appeareth to Joseph in a dream, saying, Arise, and take the young child and his mother, and flee into Egypt, and be thou there until I bring thee word: for Herod will seek the young child to destroy him."*

B. Is God telling us that he will be our partner through this process if we allow Him? God said He will make Himself know to us in a vision; Numbers 12:6 King James Version (KJV) [6]*And he said, Hear now my words: If there be a prophet among you, I the LORD will make myself known unto him in a vision, and will speak unto him in a dream.*

C. Is God telling us what type of business to start? Jacob's dream Genesis 28: 12-17 [12]*And he dreamed, and behold a ladder set up on the earth, and the top of it reached to heaven: and behold the angels of God ascending and descending on it.* [13]*And, behold, the LORD stood above it, and said, I am the LORD God of Abraham thy father, and the God of Isaac: the land whereon thou liest, to thee will I give it, and to thy seed; [14]And thy seed shall be as the dust of the earth, and thou shalt spread abroad to the west, and to the east, and to the north, and to the south: and in thee and in thy seed shall all the families of the earth be blessed. [15]And, behold, I am with thee, and will keep thee in all places whither thou goest, and will bring thee again into this land; for I will not leave thee, until I have done that which I have spoken to thee of. [16]And Jacob awaked out of his sleep, and he said, Surely the LORD is in this place; and I knew it not. [17]And he was afraid, and said, How dreadful is this place! this is none other but the house of God, and this is the gate of heaven.*

Will God give me all the gifts I need for the ministry or business He blessed me with?

God grants supernatural gifts through dreams. 1st Kings 3:5-15 [5]*At Gibeon the LORD appeared to Solomon during the night in a dream, and God said, "Ask for whatever you want me to give you."* [6]*Solomon answered, "You have shown great kindness to your servant, my father David, because he was faithful to you and righteous and upright in heart. You have continued this great kindness to him and have given him a son to sit on his throne this very day.* [7]*"Now, LORD my God, you have made your servant king in place of my father David. But I am only a little child and do not know how to carry out my duties.* [8]*Your servant is here among the people you have chosen, a great people, too*

numerous to count or number. [9]So give your servant a
discerning heart to govern your people and to distinguish
between right and wrong. For who is able to govern this
great people of yours?" [10]The Lord was pleased that
Solomon had asked for this. [11]So God said to him, "Since
you have asked for this and not for long life or wealth for
yourself, nor have asked for the death of your enemies but
for discernment in administering justice, [12]I will do what
you have asked. I will give you a wise and discerning heart,
so that there will never have been anyone like you, nor will
there ever be. [13]Moreover, I will give you what you have not
asked for—both wealth and honor—so that in your lifetime
you will have no equal among kings. [14]And if you walk in
obedience to me and keep my decrees and commands as
David your father did, I will give you a long life." [15]Then
Solomon awoke—and he realized it had been a dream.

Will God instruct us who to do business or ministry with and where to go to do business/ ministry?

Acts 16:9 King James Version (KJV) *[9]And a vision*
appeared to Paul in the night; There stood a man of
Macedonia, and prayed him, saying, Come over into
Macedonia, and help us. [10]And after he had seen the vision,
immediately we endeavoured to go into Macedonia,
assuredly gathering that the Lord had called us for to
preach the gospel unto them.

Will God warn us when we withdraw from Sunday and midweek services because we are too busy with the business He has blessed me with to serve and worship Him as we did previously?

God will show us that we are heading on a dangerous path so we can change. Job 33:14-18 King James Version (KJV)
14 *For God speaketh once, yea twice, yet man perceiveth it not.* 15 *In a dream, in a vision of the night, when deep sleep falleth upon men, in slumberings upon the bed;* 16 *Then he openeth the ears of men, and sealeth their instruction,*
17 *That he may withdraw man from his purpose, and hide pride from man.* 18 *He keepeth back his soul from the pit, and his life from perishing by the sword.*

Will God give me that last formula I need to complete the invention He down loaded to me in a dream?

For example, He established the Abrahamic Covenant in a dream; Genesis 15: 12-13 and 18 King James Version (KJV)
12 *And when the sun was going down, a deep sleep fell upon Abram; and, lo, an horror of great darkness fell upon him.*
13 *And he said unto Abram, Know of a surety that thy seed shall be a stranger in a land that is not theirs, and shall serve them; and they shall afflict them four hundred years;...* 18 *In the same day the LORD made a covenant with Abram, saying, Unto thy seed have I given this land, from the river of Egypt unto the great river, the river Euphrates:"*

Two Types of Dreams

Dreams about us

If you are an active contributor in your dream and people or things can hear you then the dream is about you.

Dreams that belong to others

If when you speak, no one can hears you and sometimes you stand above watching what's happening rather than contributing with what's going on this is a clue that the dream is about someone else. Ask God what to do with the information. Maybe you are to pray for the person you are dreaming about instead of relating it to them. **Get confirmation from Holy Spirit before informing the person about the dream.**

Thoughts

Interpreting Our Dreams

Five ways in which God helps us to interprets our dreams are as follows

God is the interpreter of dreams and visions. He gives us the interpretation of our dreams, therefore we should pray for God to assist us in interpreting our dream before we attempt to do so.

1. Sometime as we write down our dreams God will reveal the meaning
2. God sometimes reveals the meaning of a dream as he gives it to us as we are dreaming
3. God will sometimes reveal the meaning of our dreams as we matures
4. God sometimes simultaneously reveal the meaning of our dreams
5. He sometimes uses a prophet to interpret our dreams

Thoughts

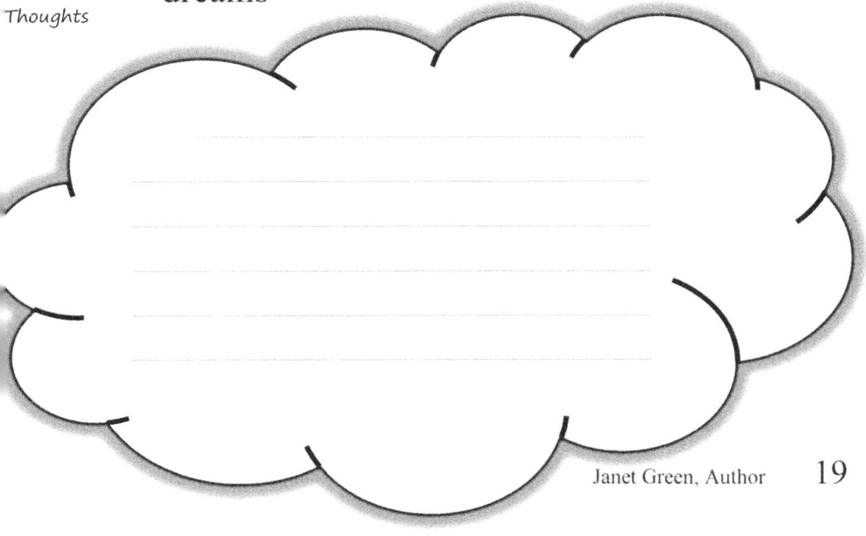

Basic things we need to know and do as God works through us to interpret our dreams

Documenting Your Dreams

- **What was your <u>Focal Emotion</u> in the dream?**
    - Your feelings during the dream.
- **What was your <u>Focal Action</u>** (Falling, Flying, Driving)?
    - Most dominant action the dream left you with
- **<u>Who was Referred</u> to in the dream?**
    - Is the dream about you or someone else?
- **What <u>Subject was your dream</u> about?**
- **What was the <u>Date and Time</u>**
    - The date and time of your dream occurs can link to *Bible* scripture or a month or date of a future event.
- **What were the <u>Symbols</u>?**
    - Symbols may come from your life/your surroundings.

Never forget to pray, ask God for His assistance in interpreting your dreams. God speaks to us in our dreams concerning our relationship with Him, our family, health, friends, foes, ministry, and our jobs. Therefore, He takes pleasure in assisting us with interpreting our dreams.

Please use dream documentation form in the back of this book.

Sample Dream 1

I was at the doctor with a group of women who were there for pregnancy tests. As I looked at my results and it showed that I was six months pregnant. I told everyone in my family. My dad asked me, "Who's the father?" I was confused because I did not have an answer. I went outside and started walking up a grassy hill.

I thought, "Was it Carl's baby?" Then I thought, "No, it couldn't have been because we had not slept together." I was wondering why God did not tell me whose baby it was and at that point, I woke from my sleep.

Sample Dream 2

I was upstairs in a large building with glass windows. A baby was running around on the floor. I took the baby and started pampering it. I lay down and started to put the baby to sleep when I heard three women start to argue and calling for me. I ignored them until I was finished taking care of the baby.

When I got up from taking care of the baby I looked through the window, they did not see me but I saw them. I asked how I could help. I do not remember how

I got to the lower level where they were but I was there with them. All three of them approach me to fight. I was very calm. I was not afraid. I tried to keep them from going behind me so I could see them all time.

One of the women asked me, "Are you 48?" I said, "No." At that point, they became quiet. They down sat in a circle. One of the women put her hand in her abdomen and pulled out everything except her heart, kidney, and liver. She asked me to select one. I said to her, "You must be crazy. I am not going to touch that mess." At this point, I awoke from my dream.

Please use dream documentation form in the back of this book.

Thoughts

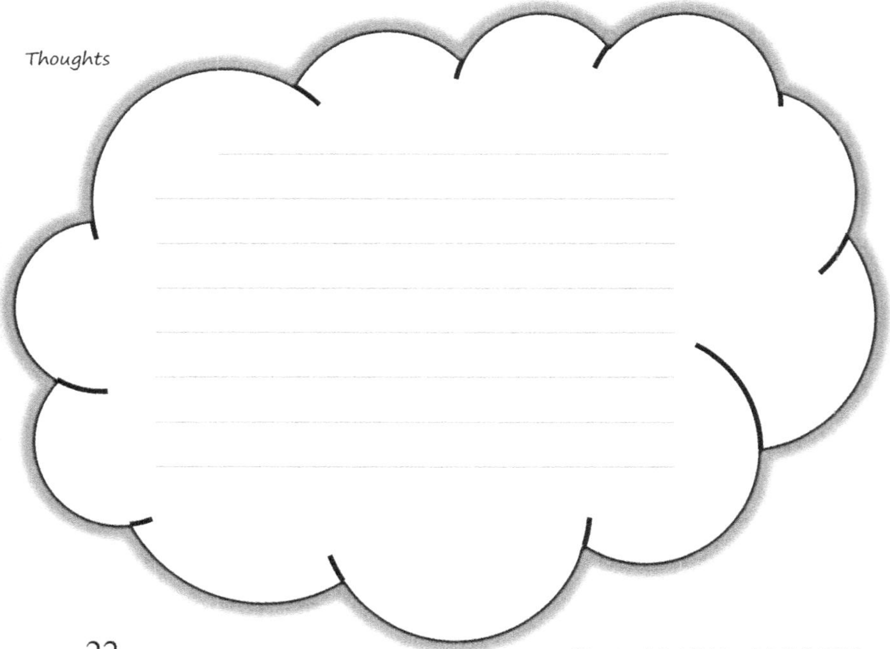

Symbols in Our Dreams

A. **Numbers**

Numbers in your dreams are literal.

B. **People**

People's names are very important, especially if stated in the dream. This might be an indication that you need to focus on the meaning of their name rather than the individual.

Seeing people that you have a relationship with in a dream may represent aspects of yourself. If you see a family member or friend in your dream, ask yourself, "What is her/is main quality?" For example, if you dream about your police officer brother, the dream could refer to your authoritative nature.

As you begin to have more and more dreams you can start to create a personalize symbol chart, this will help you with future interpretations. You will find that you are unique concerning the meaning of certain symbols. For example, in my dreams, my dad usually represents God while my mom often represents me. After a few interpretations of your dreams, you will begin to become familiar with who represents whom.

C. **Angels**
If an angel speaks to you in a dream it is literal.

D. **Animals**
An animal in your dream could refer to its emotion

Horse—Authority

Cat—Curiosity

Bull—Rage

Fox—Sneaky

Lion—Loyalty

Source Audio CD by Mark Virkler, 2011

E. **House**
Represents family, persons, and ministry (Matt. 7:24-27, II Tim. 2:20-21, Luke 11:24)

F. **House, discovering a new room**
If associated with positive feelings, a new area of life or ministry God will open or desires to open if you will only cooperate.
If associated with negative feelings, a dark part of your life the Lord wants to expose and/or heal.

G. **House, New**
New life, Change, new move of God, revival (2nd Corinthians 5:17)

H. House, old
Past, established tradition, in bad condition-our sins (Genesis 12:1)

I. **House, dilapidated, torn, hole in the roof**
Indicates a lack of spiritual covering; having an area of life in which God's protection has been withdrawn due to sin or an upcoming wrong choice.

J. Nakedness
Represents intimacy with God, standing naked before God represents surrendering to God (Gen. 3:8-11) Also means exposure.

K. Snakes, Serpents
Represent the enemy; lie, demons; bad omen; danger (Gen. 3:1, Num. 21:4-9). Wisdom (Matt 10:16).

L. Alligators
Someone with great influence has instigated an attack. It could be a generational curse.

M. Transportation
Represents the current path or direction of one's life due to decisions made; can also represent the person's life as in the common (E.) House symbol.

N. **Vehicles, multi-passenger (buses, trains, etc.)**
Same as "vehicles" above but involving a group of people such as one's family, church,

denomination, etc., (e.g. a bus wreck with injuries: warning that a specific decision or the current course will lead to bad results for the party involved).

O. **Water, rushing or fast flowing**
If associated with a positive feeling: indicates the blessing of God; the presence of the Holy Spirit. (Ezek. 47:1-9)

Thoughts

Important Facts

- Never interpret a person's dream unless the Holy Spirit leads you do so.
- **The dream came from the dreamer's heart; therefore, they have to witness to the interpretation.**
- When you have a recurring dream it's usually because you are not paying attention to what the dream is telling you, therefore pray and ask God for the interpretation
- Never make a major decision in your life based on one dream without receiving additional confirmation. When the Holy Spirit directed me to add a dream class to my entrepreneur ministry I prayed about it and weeks later a Prophet prophesied to me about it. Only when I received confirmation did I move forward with it.
- **ALWAYS** remember that you should pray and ask God for clarification if you are not sure what a dream means**. Thank God** for speaking to you through dreams and visions.
- The information in this book is to give you basic overview of how God will communicate with you more through dreams and visions. You are not a professional interpreter of dreams, yet; therefore do not claim to be one.

Activating Your Vision

Visions are *easier* to understand than dreams.

Applying the following principles to our visions will help us to manifest God's will for our lives

A. Pray and thank God, that He has chosen you to give you this vision. Ask God to give you grace and mercy as you go through the process for manifestation of this vision. You must also pray to activate your vision.
B. As you wait for God to reveal it to you stay positive, be very prayerful.
C. Prepare yourself, do not live in sin, and expect your vision to materialize.
D. Allow God to fulfill the vision in His time. Pray for God's continuous grace and mercy as you wait.
E. Do not lose faith if you think that the fulfillment of the vision is delayed. God's timing is not our timing. He is always on time.

Remember, Joseph received his vision at the age of seventeen and it did not manifest until he was thirty years old!

Continue to praise and worship God, thank Him for the manifestation of your vision. Do not be like the children of Israel who complained and lost their opportunity to enter into a land flowing with milk and honey. Let patience and faith be your guide.

Thoughts

Types of Dreams

Intercession

God is showing you something about another individual and you should pray for the person indicated. Get confirmation from God before you tell the individual about the vision.

Destiny

God is revealing plans and anointings for your life.

Chemical

Taking sleeping pills, drinking alcohol or any form of drugs before bedtime this can alter your dream.

Invention

God can give us an invention and/or new business idea in our dreams.

Curing

God can cure us of a sickness in our dreams; He can heal us as we dream about it.

Soul

Can take place when a person thinks of something or someone "too much" then it will begin to manifest in their dreams. This can cloud one's thinking to believe it's from the Devil. We have to guard our mind, soul, and body, make sure our thoughts are consistent with the Word of God.

Revelation

God will give us dreams of future event (prophecy).

Adjustment

God will reveal to us that we are heading on the wrong path of life and it is for us to make the necessary adjustment so that our life will line up with His will for our life. These dreams are conditional, if we pray and ask for repentance and change our action then God can deliver us.

Word of Knowledge

God will show us how to solve a problem through our dreams.

Direction

God will give us direction and what to do and when to it. Matthew 2: 13-14 [13]*And when they were departed, behold, the angel of the Lord appeareth to Joseph in a dream, saying, Arise, and take the young child and his mother, and flee into Egypt, and be thou there until I bring thee word: for Herod will seek the young child to destroy him.* [14]*When he arose, he took the young child and his mother by night, and departed into Egypt:*

Spiritual Warfare

Comes in the form of a nightmare, attacks against us and or others.

Fear Dreams

Comes from our own fears.

Deliverance

God removes demonic problems from us.

Demonic

Dark dreams, these dreams reveal the plan of the devil for our life.

Symbolic Meanings

Please take into consideration the context of your dream. Symbols don't always mean the same thing from dream to dream and individual to individual for example if a person who had a bad experience with dogs dream about a dog it might be a warning danger is ahead versus a person who loves dog and never had a bad experience with one the dream might be good fortune.

Symbols can have both positive and negative meanings. For example, dreaming of **money** could mean gain or loss of finances or favor. Of course, always rely on the context and your feelings during the dream. Most importantly, you need to rely on God's Holy Spirit to interpret your dreams.

Word	Meaning
Ants	Irritation, unwanted guest
Attic	History, old memories
Baby	New idea, new work, new beginning, new ministry, innocent
Balloon (Air)	Peacefully raining in the Holy Spirit
Bathroom	Cleansing of toxins
Battery	Limited power
Barefoot	Vulnerability, lack of peace
Bears	Unexpected attack
Bees	Demonic attack
Black Panther	Evil, sneaky
Blue	Communion, revelation, depression,

	sorrow, anxiety
Brown	compassion, humility, humanism
Building	Your family, church
Chariots	Something you are going to accomplish
Child	Something new
Circle	Covenant
Clothing	Mental, Anointing
Coat	Protection
Death/no blood	Something in your life will die, i.e., job, friend, marriage
Door	Opportunity
Dog	Trouble, problem; If you are a lover of dog/have a dog as a pet the dream could mean something good, protector, guard, man's best friend
Eight	New beginning (teacher)
Elephant	Wisdom, strength
Eleven	Transition, standing in the gap (prophet)
Falling	Loss of support, backsliding, trial
Fifteen	Mercy, rest
Five	Grace, redemption, anointing
Fifty	Holy Spirit, liberty, Pentecost
Flowers	Fragrance of the Lord
Flying	Rise above your situation, spiritual giftedness,
Forty	Generational, trial, testing, closing in on victory

Four	Four corners of the earth, universal, God's creative works
Fourteen	Double anointing,
Gate	A way of entrance, power, authority
Green	Conscience, growth, prosperity, envy, jealousy, pride
Gun	Powder, power
Gun (Water Gun)	Holy Spirit, cleansing
Hall	Transition
Hill	Elevation, promotion
Horn	Power, strength, defense
Horse	Power, authority
Hospital	Care
House	Dwelling place, church
Key	Authority, power to bind or to loosen, lock or unlock
Kitchen	Transformation
Knife	Skill, severing, cutting off, tongue, gossip
Mice	Demonic attack, you give the devil permission to be there, you left something unattended
Mirror	Showing you what's going on in your life
Money	Loss or gain of favor
Mother	Source, church, kindness,
Nail	Security, establish
Nakedness	Vulnerability, transparency
Nine	Judgment (evangelist)

Nose	Discernment
Office Building	Administration
One	God
One Hundred	Fullness, full measure, full reward
One Hundred Fifty-Three	Kingdom multiplication, revival
One Hundred Forty-Four	God's ultimate in creation
One Hundred Twenty	End of flesh
Oven	Testing, judgment
Pigs	Unclean, lead to destruction
Platter	Spiritual food coming
Purple	Authority, royalty-false authority
Purse	Issues of life, identity
Rainbow	Conversant, protection
Rat	Demonic attack, you have given the devil permission to be there.
Red	Wisdom, anointing, power-anger, war
Ribbon	Reminder
River	Move of God
Roach	Evil, something you left unattended
Roller Coaster	Instability
Roof	Covering, oversight
Seven	Perfection, completion, fullness
Seventeen	Elect of God
Six	Man, humanity, carnal
Sixteen	Established new beginnings
Snake (Long Tail)	Lie—wisdom

Snake (Short Tail)	Gossip
Spider	Occult
Sword	Word of God, ability
Teeth	Ability to think
Ten	Journey, wilderness, (pastor)
Thirteen	Rebellion
Thirty	Begin ministry
Thirty Seven	First born
Three	God Will
Transportation	Level of work, ministry, job
Tree	Leader, leadership
Turkey	Wisdom or foolishness
Twelve	Government (apostle)
Twenty Five	Begin ministry training
Two	Multiplication, division
Wall	Obstacle, barrier,
White	Spirit of the Lord, holy power,
Wind	Holy Spirit
Window	Reveal, prophecy, revelation
Yellow	Mind, hope, gift of God, fear, coward, marriage, light
	Source: Some of the dream symbols meanings came from a CD by John Paul Jackson

Exercise

Dream 1

I was at the doctor with a group of women who were there for pregnancy tests. As I looked at my results and it showed that I was six months pregnant. I told everyone in my family. My dad asked me, "Who's the father?" I was confused because I did not have an answer. I went outside and started walking up a grassy hill.

I thought, "Was it Carl's baby?" Then I thought, "No, it couldn't have been because we had not slept together." I was wondering why God did not tell me whose baby it was and at that point, I woke from my sleep.

Thoughts

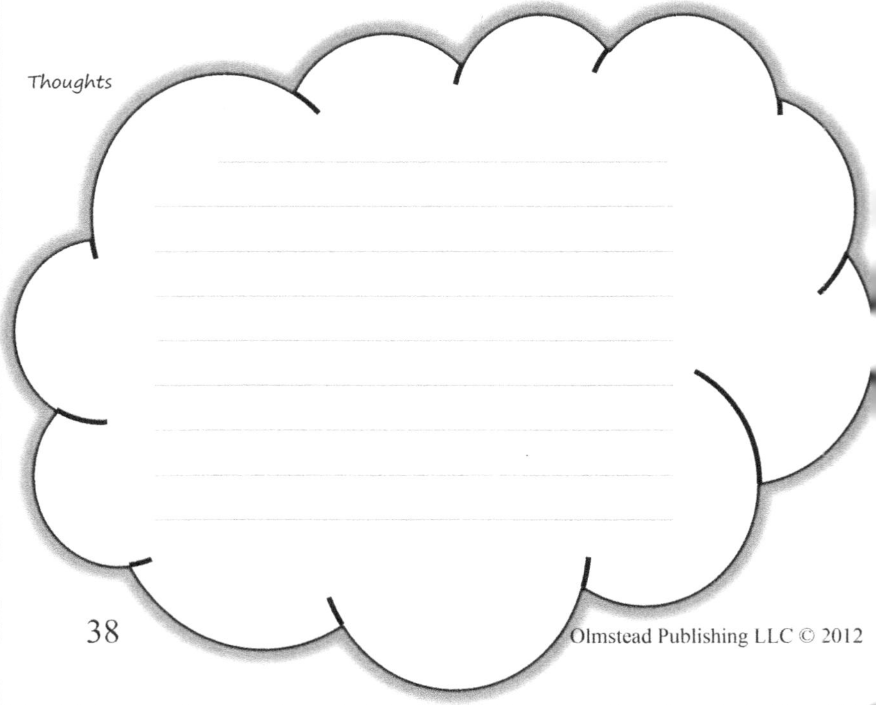

Dream 2

I was upstairs in a large building with glass windows. A baby was running around on the floor. I took the baby and started pampering it. I laid down and started to put the baby to sleep when I heard three ladies start to argue and asking for me. I ignored them until I was finished taking care of the baby.

When I got up from taking care of the baby I looked through the window, they did not see me but I saw them. I asked how I could help. I do not remember how I got to the lower level where they were but I was there with them. All three of them approach me to fight. I was very calm. I was not afraid. I tried to keep them from going behind me so I could see them all time.

One of the women asked me, "Are you 48?" I said, "No." At that point, they became quiet. They down sat in a circle. One of the women put her hand in her abdomen and pulled out everything except her heart, kidney, and liver. She asked me to select one. I said to her, "You must be crazy. I am not going to touch that mess." At this point, I awoke from my dream.

Dream Interpretation Form 1

Remember: Dreams are symbolic while visions are literal!

Title of Dream/Vision: ______________________

____

Date: ____________ **Time**: ___________

Symbol
(Personalized symbol)

Meaning

___________ ____________________________

___________ ____________________________

___________ ____________________________

___________ ____________________________

___________ ____________________________

___________ ____________________________

___________ ____________________________

___________ ____________________________

___________ ____________________________

Focal Emotion **Meaning**

(Where in my life am I experiencing this emotion)

________________ ____

________________ ____

________________ ____

________________ ____

Focal Action **Meaning**

________________ ____

________________ ____

________________ ____

________________ ____

Color **Meaning**

________________ ____

________________ ____

________________ ____

________________ ____

Dream Interpretation Form 2

Remember: Dreams are symbolic while visions are literal!

Title of Dream/Vision: ______________________

____

Date: ____________ **Time**: ___________

Symbol (Personalized symbol)	**Meaning**
___________	____________________________
___________	____________________________
___________	____________________________
___________	____________________________
___________	____________________________
___________	____________________________
___________	____________________________
___________	____________________________
___________	____________________________

Focal Emotion **Meaning**

(Where in my life am I experiencing this emotion)

Focal Action **Meaning**

Color **Meaning**

Dream Interpretation Form 3

Remember: Dreams are symbolic while visions are literal!

Title of Dream/Vision: ______________________

____

Date: ____________ **Time:** ___________

Symbol

(Personalized symbol)

Meaning

___________ ____________________________

___________ ____________________________

___________ ____________________________

___________ ____________________________

___________ ____________________________

___________ ____________________________

___________ ____________________________

___________ ____________________________

___________ ____________________________

Focal Emotion **Meaning**

(Where in my life am I experiencing this emotion)

Focal Action **Meaning**

Color **Meaning**

Dream Interpretation Form 4

Remember: Dreams are symbolic while visions are literal!

Title of Dream/Vision: ______________________

____

Date: ____________ **Time:** ___________

Symbol (Personalized symbol)	**Meaning**
___________	___________________________
___________	___________________________
___________	___________________________
___________	___________________________
___________	___________________________
___________	___________________________
___________	___________________________
___________	___________________________
___________	___________________________

Focal Emotion **Meaning**

(Where in my life am I experiencing this emotion)

Focal Action **Meaning**

Color **Meaning**

Dream Interpretation Form 5

Remember: Dreams are symbolic while visions are literal!

Title of Dream/Vision: ______________________________

____

Date: ________________ **Time**: _______________

Symbol (Personalized symbol) | **Meaning**

_______________ ______________________________________

_______________ ______________________________________

_______________ ______________________________________

_______________ ______________________________________

_______________ ______________________________________

_______________ ______________________________________

_______________ ______________________________________

_______________ ______________________________________

_______________ ______________________________________

Focal Emotion **Meaning**

(Where in my life am I experiencing this emotion)

______________ ________________________________

______________ ________________________________

______________ ________________________________

______________ ________________________________

Focal Action **Meaning**

______________ ________________________________

______________ ________________________________

______________ ________________________________

______________ ________________________________

Color **Meaning**

______________ ________________________________

______________ ________________________________

______________ ________________________________

______________ ________________________________

Dream Interpretation Form 6

Remember: Dreams are symbolic while visions are literal!

Title of Dream/Vision: ______________________

____

Date: ____________ **Time:** ___________

Symbol (Personalized symbol)	**Meaning**
___________	____________________________
___________	____________________________
___________	____________________________
___________	____________________________
___________	____________________________
___________	____________________________
___________	____________________________
___________	____________________________
___________	____________________________

Focal Emotion **Meaning**

(Where in my life am I experiencing this emotion)

Focal Action **Meaning**

Color **Meaning**

Dream Interpretation Form 7

Remember: Dreams are symbolic while visions are literal!

Title of Dream/Vision: ______________________

____

Date: ____________ **Time:** ___________

Symbol (Personalized symbol)	**Meaning**
___________	____________________________
___________	____________________________
___________	____________________________
___________	____________________________
___________	____________________________
___________	____________________________
___________	____________________________
___________	____________________________
___________	____________________________

Focal Emotion — Meaning

(Where in my life am I experiencing this emotion)

Focal Emotion	Meaning
____________	______________________________
____________	______________________________
____________	______________________________
____________	______________________________

Focal Action — Meaning

Focal Action	Meaning
____________	______________________________
____________	______________________________
____________	______________________________
____________	______________________________

Color — Meaning

Color	Meaning
____________	______________________________
____________	______________________________
____________	______________________________
____________	______________________________

Dream Interpretation Form 8

Remember: Dreams are symbolic while visions are literal!

Title of Dream/Vision: ____________________

____

Date: ____________ **Time:** ____________

Symbol (Personalized symbol)	**Meaning**
____________	______________________________
____________	______________________________
____________	______________________________
____________	______________________________
____________	______________________________
____________	______________________________
____________	______________________________
____________	______________________________
____________	______________________________

Focal Emotion **Meaning**

(Where in my life am I experiencing this emotion)

Focal Action **Meaning**

Color **Meaning**

Author

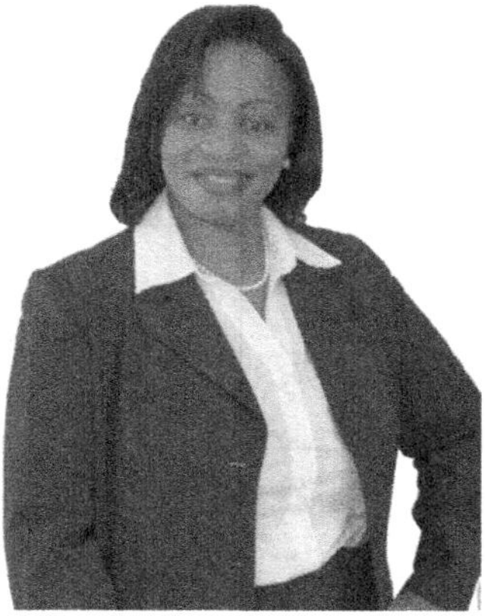

Janet Green, the proud mother of three young men of God, created "God's Will Ministry." As a Director of New Destiny Christian Center Entrepreneur Ministry, she teaches people how to start a business. She volunteered as an ambassador for three different Chambers of Commerce in central Florida namely; Central Florida Christian Chamber of Commerce, Apopka Chamber of Commerce, and the African American Chamber of Commerce.

Janet now speaks in prisons, evangelizes in her church community, and visits a local hospital on weekends where she prays for the sick. Janet is frequently interviewed about her latest books **Dream and Visions from God** or **How to Turn Your Talent into a Business**. As if this does not keep her busy enough, she cooks and serves the homeless.

At age 14, Janet had her first experience in business leadership when she helped her Uncle Gigi manage his poultry business. Her 20-year career in the hospitality industry began in New York City as a hotel PBX operator and ended as a Director of Human Resources.

janet@godwills.com
www.facebook.com/GodSpeaksToUsThroughDreamsAndVisions
www.facebook.com/Talent2business

- Through God ALL things are possible.
- Ask and it will be done.
- Seek and ye shall find.

Made in the USA
Monee, IL
04 November 2026

67382341R00036